MUSTARD

MARIAN KIM

ISBN: 1508665974

ISBN-13: 978-1508665977

CONTENTS

1

PROPERTIES

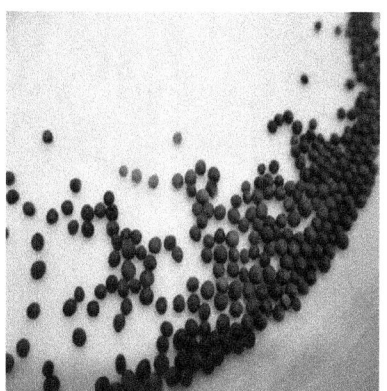

Scientific name: Brassica nigra

Other names: Black moutarde, sinapis nigra

Nutrients: Omega 3 fatty acids, calcium, iron, magnesium, manganese, phosphorous, selenium, zinc

Properties

Anti-cancer properties

Analgesic (pain relieving) properties

Antiseptic (antibacterial, antifungal) properties

Antioxidant properties which protect the cells from the free radical damage that causes premature aging and degenerative disease

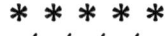

2

USES

Coughs, pneumonia and bronchitis treatment

Mustard poultices and mustard plasters are used to treat coughs, chest congestion, pneumonia, bronchitis and pleurisy. They improve blood circulation and their aroma also clears up the congestion.

A mustard footbath can also be used to relieve chest congestion.

Common cold and flu

Black mustard oil is used for the common cold. Mustard plasters are also used to relieve congestion associated with these conditions. Mustard baths are also used to relieve the symptoms of colds.

Arthritis treatment

Mustard plasters are used to treat arthritis and joint aches. Black mustard oil is also used for arthritis and rheumatism. It is usually applied when warm. Mustard infused oils and salves can also be used to treat aching joints.

Muscle ache relief

Mustard plasters are used to treat muscle aches and lumbago (lower back pain) since they relieve the pain and loosen stiff muscles. Mustard baths are also used to relieve tired and aching muscles.

Weight loss

Mustard seeds increase the body's metabolism helping it burn more calories. Therefore consider adding half a teaspoon of mustard seeds to your diet each day since this can help you burn more calories even when you are resting.

Digestive aid

Mustard stimulates the appetite and increases the flow of saliva and other digestive juices.

Edema treatment

Black mustard seed is used for edema (water retention).

Anorexia

Black mustard seed is used for anorexia to increase the appetite.

Emesis

Black mustard seed is used to cause vomiting.

Diuresis

Black mustard seed is used diuresis (increase urine production).

Aching feet

Mustard poultice can be applied to aching feet to relieve the pain. A mustard foot bath can also be used for the same purpose.

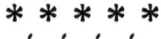

3

SAFETY PRECAUTIONS

1. Consuming large amounts of black mustard seed orally (by mouth) can injure the throat and cause heart failure, diarrhea, drowsiness, difficulties breathing, coma and death.

2. Applying black mustard seed to the skin for a long time can cause blisters.

3. Women who are pregnant should not use black mustard seed since it can cause miscarriages.

4

DRUG INTERACTIONS

None known todate.

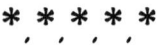

5

HERBAL RECIPES

Mustard Poultice

Equipment

Cheesecloth or old cotton sheet strips

***

Ingredients

¼ cup Mustard powder

¼ cup Bran

Boiling water

***

Instructions

1. Add enough boiling water to the mustard and bran to wet it and make a thick paste.

2. Spoon the mustard paste onto the cheesecloth (or bed sheet strips) to make the poultice.

3. To use, apply the poultice to the affected area and cover with another piece of hot, wet cloth. Replace the hot, wet cloth when it cools with another hot one to keep the poultice hot.

*****

Mustard Plaster

Equipment

Cotton handkerchief or old cotton sheet squares

***

Ingredients

1 tablespoon Mustard powder

3 tablespoons Whole wheat flour (use 6 tablespoons if making plasters for children)

Hot water

***

Instructions

1. Add enough hot water to the mustard and wheat flour to wet it and make a spreadable paste.

2. Spoon the mustard and flour paste onto the handkerchief (or bed sheet square) to make the poultice.

3. To use, apply the plaster to the affected area and cover with another piece of hot, wet cloth. A heavy blanket can also be placed on top of the plaster to encourage sweating.

4. Remove the plaster from the chest after 15 minutes.

5. Another mustard plaster can also be prepared for the back.

***

Tips

1. Mustard plasters should not be left on the skin for more than 15 minutes since they can burn the skin and cause blisters. After they are

removed the skin should be washed with warm water and a layer of Vaseline applied.

*****

Mustard Bath

Equipment

Wide mouthed jar with air tight lid

***

Ingredients

1 cup baking soda

4 tablespoons mustard powder

10 drops essential oils like eucalyptus or peppermint

***

Instructions

1. Mix all the ingredients in the jar with the air tight lid.

2. To use, add 2 tablespoons of the mixture into a bathtub filled with warm water.

*****

Mustard Footbath

Equipment

Foot bath or bowl large enough to soak feet

***

Ingredients

1 tablespoon mustard powder

1 quart (1000 ml) hot water

***

Instructions

1. Put the mustard to the hot water.

2. Let the water cool before soaking feet in it.

***

Tips

1. Add 1 teaspoon of ginger to the mustard footbath to make it more potent for relieving aching feet.

*****

Mustard Infused Oil

Equipment

Double boiler

Large glass bowl

Sieve and cheesecloth

Sterilized dark jars

***

Ingredients

16 fl oz. (500 ml) vegetable oil like organic olive, sweet almond oil or sunflower oil

8 oz. (250 grams) mustard

***

Instructions

1. Place the mustard and oil in the glass bowl ensuring that the oil covers the mustard. Simmer them in a double boiler for one hour at a temperature of around 120 degrees Fahrenheit (49 degrees Celsius). Do not let the mixture boil. You can repeat this step several times after letting the oils cool to create more concentrated herb infused oils.

2. Strain the mixture through the sieve and cheesecloth into a clean, dark jar ensuring you squeeze out as much oil as you can from the cheesecloth.

3. Label your jars with the manufacturing date, expiry date, mustard and oils used.

4. Store your mustard infused oils in a cool dark place or in the refrigerator and use them within 3 months.

*****

Mustard Salve

Equipment

Double boiler

Large glass bowl

Sterilized dark jars or tins

***

Ingredients

8 oz. (250 ml or 1 cup) mustard infused vegetable oil (see previous recipe)

1 oz. (30 grams) beeswax

10 drops essential oils like lavender essential oil (optional natural fragrance)

***

Instructions

1. Place the beeswax and mustard infused oil in the glass bowl and melt them in a double boiler.

2. Once melted remove from the heat source, allow to cool and add the essential oils (if using).

3. Pour the melted oils into the storage jars or tins and allow to cool completely.

4. Store the salves in a cool dark place.

###

ABOUT THE AUTHOR

Marian Kim is an experienced alternative medicine practitioner.

*****

OTHER BOOKS BY THE AUTHOR

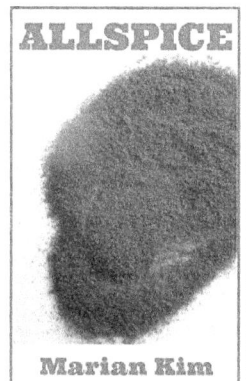

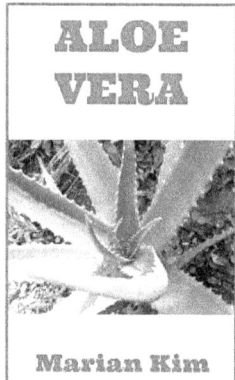

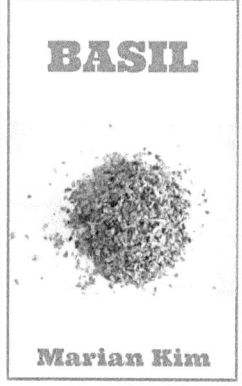

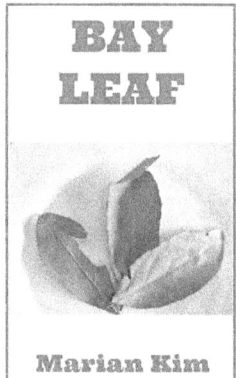

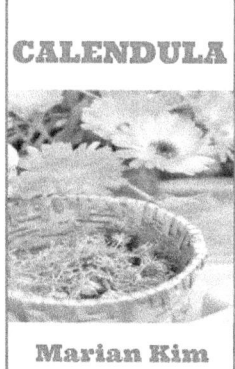

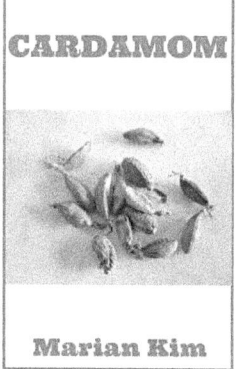

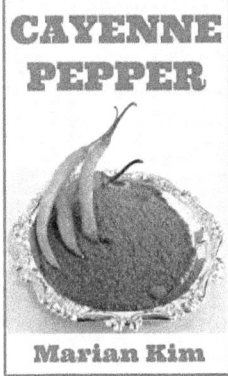

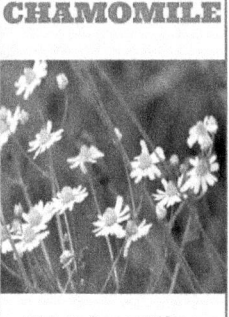

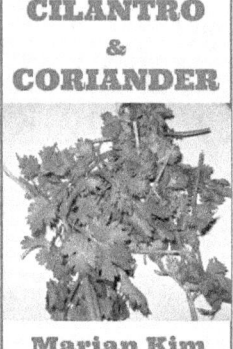

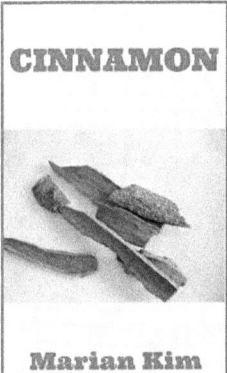

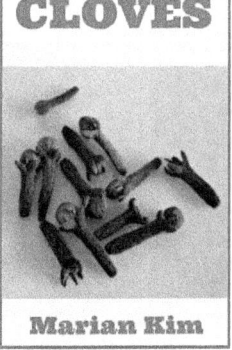

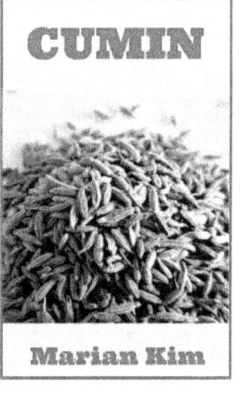

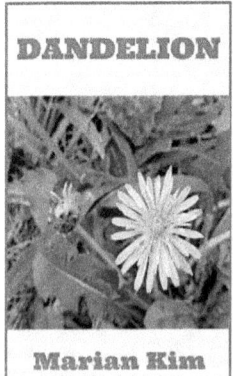

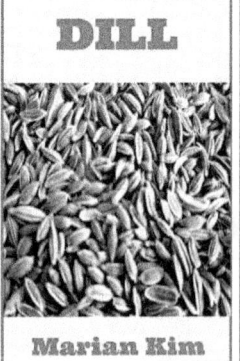

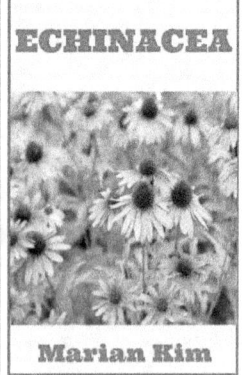

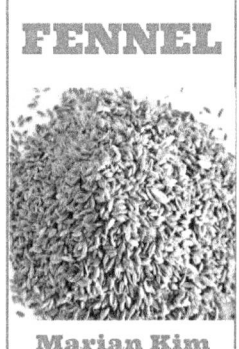

FENNEL

Marian Kim

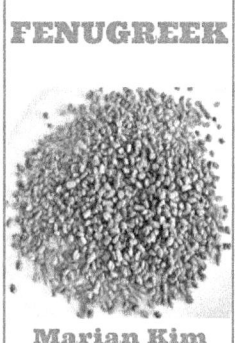

FENUGREEK

Marian Kim

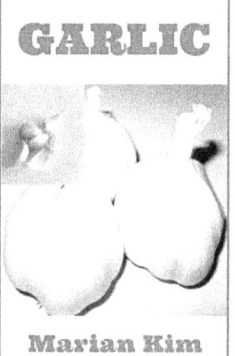

GARLIC

Marian Kim

GINGER

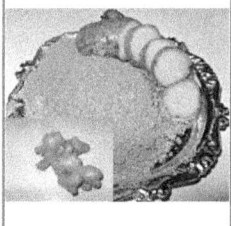

Marian Kim

GINKGO BILOBA

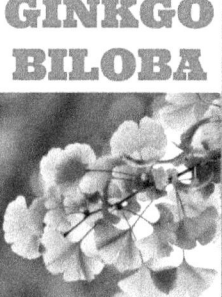

Marian Kim

GINSENG

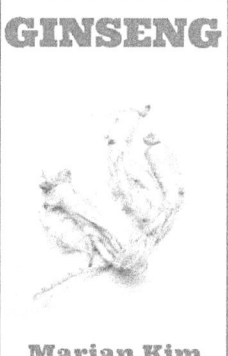

Marian Kim

LAVENDER

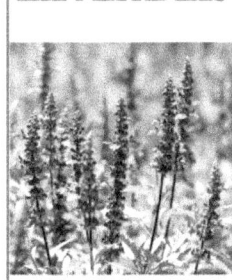

Marian Kim

MUSTARD

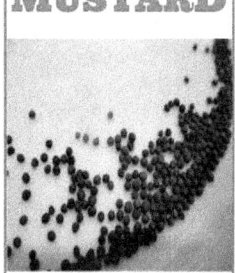

Marian Kim

NEEM

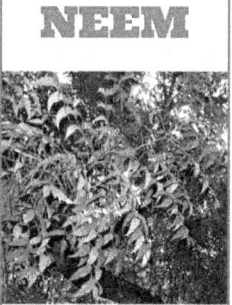

Marian Kim

NUTMEG & MACE
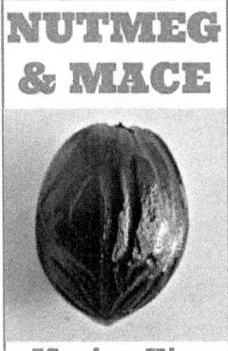
Marian Kim

OREGANO
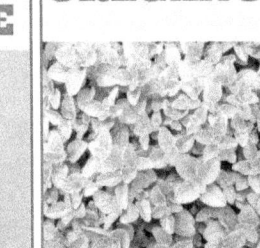
Marian Kim

PAPRIKA

Marian Kim

PARSLEY
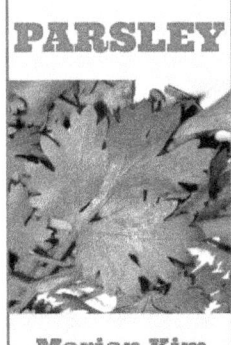
Marian Kim

BLACK & WHITE PEPPER
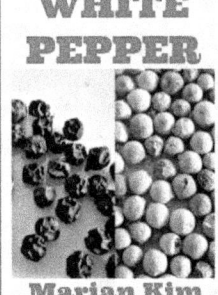
Marian Kim

PEPPERMINT
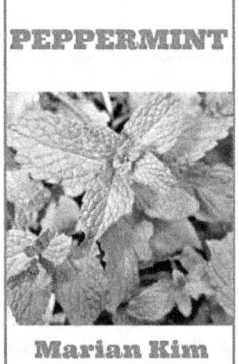
Marian Kim

ROSE HIPS
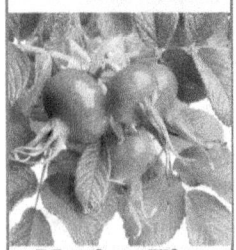
Marian Kim

ROSE PETALS

Marian Kim

ROSEMARY
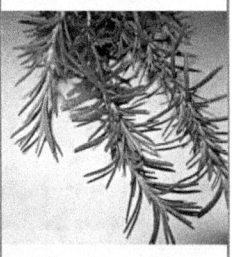
Marian Kim

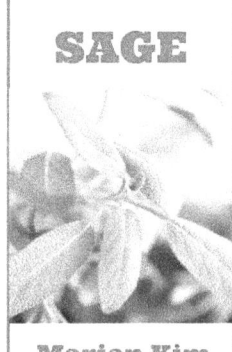

SAGE

Marian Kim

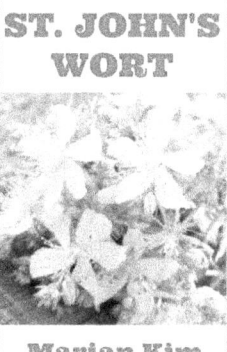

ST. JOHN'S WORT

Marian Kim

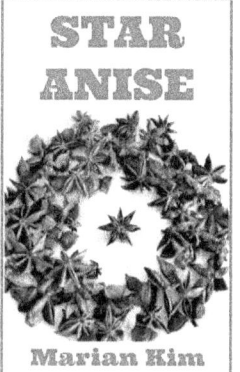

STAR ANISE

Marian Kim

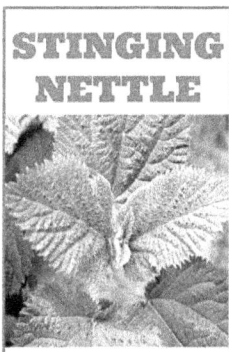

STINGING NETTLE

Marian Kim

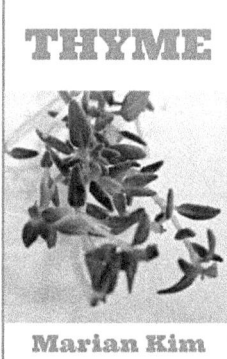

THYME

Marian Kim

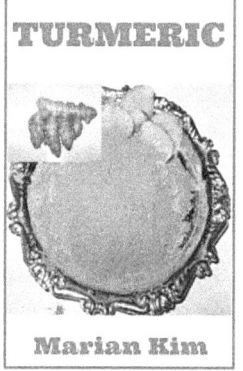

TURMERIC

Marian Kim

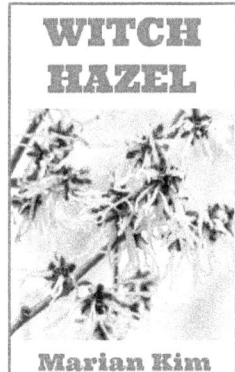

WITCH HAZEL

Marian Kim

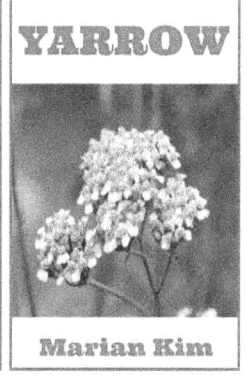

YARROW

Marian Kim

*****